Everything You Need To Know About Vitamin C

Just the Facts

Guang Kao

Copyright © 2024 by Guang Kao

Disclaimer

The information provided in this book is for educational and informational purposes only. It is not intended as a substitute for professional medical advice, diagnosis, or treatment. Always seek the advice of your physician or other qualified health provider with any questions you may have regarding a medical condition.

The author and publisher do not endorse any specific product or service mentioned in this book.

While every effort has been made to ensure the accuracy of the information presented, the rapid and ever-changing nature of health and nutrition research means that information may become outdated. The author and publisher are not responsible for any errors or omissions or for the results obtained from the use of this information.

TABLE OF CONTENT

INTRODUCTION

Welcome to the world of Vitamin C

Vitamin C refers to a collection of water-soluble compounds (ascorbic acid, L-ascorbic acid, ascorbate, L-ascorbate). Few nutrients have gotten as much attention and respect in the world of health and wellbeing as Vitamin C. Vitamin C is widely regarded as a vital component of human well-being due to its high antioxidant effects and critical role in sustaining good health. Vitamin C is an essential vitamin that is involved in many physiological processes in the human body, including tissue development and maintenance, oxidative stress reduction, immunological control, and many other metabolic activities. It also participates in the synthesis of essential chemicals such as catecholamines and vasopressin. Vitamin C deficiency has been linked to a wide range of illnesses, including neoplasia, endocrinopathies, and neurologic problems. It may be related to increased disease severity and lower survival in critically sick human patients.

At its foundation, Vitamin C acts as a guardian, protecting our bodies from the onslaught of damaging free radicals. These minuscule nuisances are caused by stress, pollution, and even the act of breathing. In this scenario, however, Vitamin C emerges as a tenacious guardian, contributing electrons to neutralize free radicals and prevent cellular damage. It's a delicate dance between nature's components, and Vitamin C expertly orchestrates it.

Vitamin C forms the very fibers of our physical being, in addition to its antioxidant properties. This unassuming vitamin is responsible for much of the structure and suppleness of our skin, bones, and blood vessels. Vitamin C stimulates collagen formation through a finely organized set of reactions, ensuring the durability of our skin and the integrity of our connective tissues. It is not merely an unseen power in our world; it is the architect of our structural strength.

As we go deeper into the world of Vitamin C, we discover its synergistic relationship with our immune system. It is a protector who fortifies our immune cells, allowing them to establish a firm fight against diseases and illnesses. As we go through this world, we realize that Vitamin C is more than just a supplement; it is a sentinel of wellness, protecting us from invisible hazards.

So, welcome to the world of vitamin C. A world where science and nature coexist, where health and vitality are intertwined. As we travel through this terrain, we observe the intricate mechanics and bask in the glow of its potential, and also harness its advantages for a life that is not only healthy, but lively. This world invites us to take a step ahead, to immerse ourselves in the glories of Vitamin C, and to discover the secrets it contains for our well-being.

Why Vitamin C is vital for your health

According to epidemiological research, hypovitaminosis C remains quite frequent in Western countries, and vitamin C insufficiency is the fourth leading nutritional shortfall in the United States.

Reduced consumption paired with restricted bodily storage are among the reasons. Increased requirements are caused by pollution and smoking, as well as battling infections and disorders with oxidative and inflammatory components, such as type 2 diabetes. Adequate vitamin C consumption, either through food or supplementation, is essential for good immune function and infection resistance, particularly in groups such as the elderly or those exposed to risk factors for vitamin C deficiency. Vitamin C may help to prevent or reduce the risk of certain chronic diseases. Eating high-vitamin C foods, such as fruits and vegetables, may lower your chance of getting lung, breast, and colon cancers, as well as cardiovascular disease, according to the National Institutes of Health. Vitamin C may even lower your chances of acquiring age-related macular degeneration (AMD) and cataracts. There is some evidence that consuming vitamin C may assist persons with hypertension to decrease their blood pressure.

Vitamin C is an antioxidant, which means that it is one of several natural compounds that may aid in the treatment, slowing, or prevention of certain health conditions. It accomplishes this by neutralizing free radicals, which are unstable chemicals capable of causing cell damage and illness.

Vitamin C is believed to aid in the absorption of some nutrients, such as iron. The most well-known application of vitamin C is to improve the immune system. The antioxidant action of vitamin C may be beneficial to brain function. Vitamin C may possibly help treat or reduce your risk of mental health illnesses such as depression and anxiety.

These are among many other benefits and reasons why Vitamin C is vital for our health, as we delve deeper into consequent chapters and sub topics we will see many other vital importance of Vitamin C to our health.

How this book will guide you to understand the facts about Vitamin C

The book's core theme is the investigation of the different health advantages connected with Vitamin C.

Readers are provided with evidence-based perspectives about Vitamin C functions throughout the body, providing light on its position as a powerful antioxidant, immune system booster, and collagen production promoter with scientific basis that helps readers to comprehend the fundamental mechanisms underpinning Vitamin C's numerous advantages.

This book is a valuable resource for anyone who wants to learn more about Vitamin C and its importance. The book's well researched material gives a thorough analysis of numerous elements relating to this crucial nutrient. Furthermore, the book explains the sources of Vitamin C and its dietary needs, allowing readers to make informed decisions about incorporating this nutrient into their everyday life.

The book also educates readers with practical information to enhance their health and well-being by addressing concerns such as recommended daily consumption, dietary sources rich in Vitamin C, and probable side effects and deficiency symptoms.

By providing evidence-based insights, the book encourages readers to make educated health decisions and consider Vitamin C as an important component of their wellness regimen. This resource is important in developing educated personal health and wellness decisions, eventually directing readers toward a better and more informed healthy lifestyle.

So Enjoy !

Chapter 1

The Basics of Vitamin C

What is Vitamin C?

Vitamin C is a water-soluble vitamin that is found largely in the body in its reduced form, Ascorbic acid, and this is because it is rapidly converted intracellularly to ascorbic acid. The oxidized form of vitamin C, dehydroascorbic acid (DHA), also possesses an antiscorbutic (scurvy-preventive) effect.

Humans and other primates cannot produce vitamin C (Ascorbic Acid), the antiscorbutic vitamin, and must acquire it from food. Ascorbic acid is a cofactor for fifteen mammalian enzymes and an electron donor. Ascorbic acid is carried by two sodium-dependent transporters, whereas its oxidation product dehydroascorbic acid is delivered by glucose transporters.

Most tissues and bodily fluids collect ascorbic acid differently. The concentrations of vitamin C in plasma and tissues are affected by the amount taken, bioavailability, renal excretion, and utilization.

Vitamin C, on the other hand, is generated by all plants and most animals. It is a vitamin for humans since the gene for gulonolactone oxidase, the terminal enzyme in the Ascorbic Acid manufacturing pathway, has been mutated, rendering it inactive. Because of evidence that oxidative damage is a root cause of, or at least related with, many illnesses, there is a lot of interest in the therapeutic functions of vitamin C.

In order to be biologically meaningful or therapeutically relevant, in vitro and in vivo investigations of vitamin C activities must account for physiologic vitamin concentrations. The vitamin C is largely delivered into cells as DHA and is converted intracellularly to ascorbic acid. Because the vitamin's metabolism is controlled by many systems, little quantities are retained, while large levels are tolerated without harmful consequences. A dose-dependent active transport pathway regulates ascorbic acid absorption in the intestine. Absorption is around 70-90% at dietary doses of 30-180 mg per day, and less than 50% at intakes larger than 1g per day. However when vitamin C consumption is less than 100 mg per day, absorption is efficient, and little or no ascorbate is eliminated in the urine.

Because the oxidized or spent form of the vitamin is easily converted back to ascorbic acid, very little quantities are lost by catabolism (5-45 mg per day). At higher doses, absorption becomes less effective, and unmetabolized ascorbic acid is eliminated in the urine. The capacity of the vitamin to give electrons and be rapidly converted back to its reduced state by glutathione accounts for its unique efficiency as an in vivo antioxidant.

The total vitamin content of the human body ranges from 300 mg near scurvy to a high of about 2 grams. The concentration of the vitamin in bodily tissues and fluids varies widely, with high amounts maintained in leukocytes, eyes, adrenals, pituitary, and brain, and low levels found in plasma and saliva.

Historical background and discovery

Scurvy has been recognized since ancient times, although it only became a significant cause of large-scale fatalities in the last 500 years. Scurvy affected major land armies and cities in Northern Europe, particularly during the winter and siege warfare. Scurvy became the primary issue restricting sea voyages throughout the period of discovery, typically killing many sailors after 2 to 3 months at sea.

James Lind demonstrated that citrus fruits may heal scurvy in what was possibly the first controlled clinical experiment. However, for several decades, this easy cure was not widely employed. The discovery contradicted current scientific knowledge, and prevailing theories of illness made no mention of nutritional inadequacy.

Albert Szent-Gyorgyi discovered ascorbic acid in 1928, and SzentGyorgyi and King demonstrated it to be an antiscorbutic factor in 1932.

Functions and benefits of Vitamin C

Protection Against Oxidative Stress

During oxidative stress situations, nitric oxide (NO) depletion and the production of reactive oxygen species (ROS) are major causes of vascular dysfunction and tissue damage. Oxidative stress has been linked to aging, numerous chronic disorders, and systemic assaults such as sepsis. The impact of oxidative stress on the body might range from subclinical harm to severe organ malfunction and failure. Nitric Oxide deficiency causes vasoconstriction of terminal arterioles, whereas Reactive Oxygen Species generates a prothrombotic condition, resulting in the production of microthrombi. These alterations result in lower capillary perfusion and, as a result, decreased tissue oxygen supply. Production of ROS is frequently related to reduced NO production.

Superoxide and other ROS will be scavenged by vitamin C, which will otherwise combine with NO to generate the extremely reactive free radical peroxynitrite, which causes direct damage to proteins, lipids, and DNA. This way, ascorbate reduces the oxidation products generated by peroxynitrite interactions with cell proteins and thereby protects the body from oxidative stress.

Cancer Prevention

Both cancer development and growth of tumors include free radicals and oxidative mechanisms. Ascorbic acid, as an antioxidant, may inhibit several of these activities. Furthermore, ascorbic acid suppresses the synthesis of carcinogenic nitrosamines from dietary precursors by functioning as a nitrite trap.

Cardiovascular Risk Reduction

Ascorbic acid, like other antioxidants, may help to prevent atherogenesis by inhibiting the conversion of low-density lipoprotein (LDL) to its more atherogenic oxidized form. Several studies have found that higher ascorbic acid intakes or plasma levels are related to reduced blood pressure. Various studies have also observed blood pressure reductions of 4-11% over a wide range of plasma ascorbic acid levels

Prevention of Cataract

Cataracts are caused in part by oxidative damage to lens proteins. Antioxidant substances, like vitamin C, may help to postpone or prevent the formation of cataracts.

Capillary Perfusion

Vitamin C enhances blood flow distribution by restoring the production of Nitric Oxide (NO) by Nitric Oxide production (NOS). It may also limit the production and activity of NADPH oxidases (Nox), boosting NO levels and encouraging anti-aggregation in prothrombotic conditions. Vitamin C and hydrocortisone have been proven in vitro to work synergistically in protecting vascular endothelium against endotoxin damage. These processes may explain vitamin C's usefulness in sustaining capillary perfusion as well as decreasing vascular permeability and edema production in critically sick individuals.

Catecholamine Synthesis

Catecholamines regulate cardiovascular responses, neurotransmission, and fight or flight reactions. Vitamin C is crucial in tissues because it is necessary for two enzymatic stages in the catecholamine biosynthesis pathway. It is a cofactor for the enzyme dopamine b-hydroxylase, which converts dopamine to norepinephrine. Furthermore, vitamin C speeds up the rate-limiting phase by recycling the enzyme cofactor to create the dopamine precursor L-DOPA. In patients with vasoplegic shock, parenteral vitamin C administration may boost catecholamine production, resulting in decreased exogenous catecholamine needs. Vitamin C has also been proven to promote alpha and beta-adrenergic receptor function by attaching to the receptor and allowing for better epinephrine activation.

Vasopressin Synthesis

Vitamin C is also required for the formation of vasopressin. Arginine vasopressin (AVP) or antidiuretic hormone (ADH) is a peptide hormone generated in the brain and stored as a mature hormone in the posterior pituitary. In response to decreased circulating blood volume, decreased arterial pressure, or increased plasma osmolality, the hormone is produced, resulting in vasoconstriction, increased water retention, and adrenocorticotropic hormone (ACTH) production. Vitamin C functions as a cofactor for the enzyme peptidylglycine a-amidating monooxygenase (PAM), which is essential for vasopressin production. As a result, systemic vitamin C levels may influence the quantity of vasopressin production. This was proven in a rat research where centrally given vitamin C increased circulation vasopressin levels and promoted antidiuresis.

Immune Function

Vitamin C concentrations in immune and inflammatory cells are generally 50-to 100-fold greater than in plasma. This is most likely owing to the cells' oxidative stress and exposure to elevated Reactive Oxygen Species (ROS) concentrations during inflammatory processes. Vitamin C has been demonstrated to boost chemotaxis and phagocytosis, increase lymphocyte proliferation, and aid in oxidative neutrophilic bacterial death. Furthermore, vitamin C modulates the production of pro-inflammatory and anti-inflammatory cytokines, influences natural killer (NK) cell killing of bacteria, and decreases cytotoxic T cell activity.

Recommended Daily Intake

The daily need for vitamin C to avoid scurvy is roughly 10 mg. The former RDA for vitamin C, 60 mg per day for adults, sought to produce a whole body pool of ascorbate (e.g., 900-1,500 mg) that avoided scurvy for many weeks when low vitamin C consumption, and periods of physiologic or other stress may raise the needs. The revised RDA for vitamin C has been set at 75 mg per day for females and 90 mg per day for males to offer antioxidant protection.

The RDA for vitamin C is 60 mg per day, based on threshold urine excretion of the vitamin and avoiding the vitamin C deficient illness scurvy with a margin of safety.

If vitamin C consumption was discontinued, a daily dose of 60mg was suggested to avoid scurvy for 30-45 days. The 60-mg daily dosage was shown to cause threshold urine excretion of vitamin C. At 60 mg, tissue reserves were assumed to be near saturation, and greater doses would result in increasing excretion.

In the United States and Canada, the recommended daily amount (RDA) for vitamin C is 75 mg for women and 90 mg for men. In recent years, several nations have raised their RDAs for vitamin C to levels comparable to or somewhat higher than those in the United States and Canada.
An ideal RDA should be based on a consumption that promotes optimal health rather than simply preventing deficiencies.

A daily intake of five servings of fruits and vegetables will supply enough levels of vitamin C (about 200-250 mg of vitamin C).

The RDAs from 1989 advised that habitual cigarette smokers should consume at least 100 mg of vitamin C each day. Because of the increased oxidative stress induced by cigarette smoking, cigarette smokers may require an additional 16 mg of vitamin C for every pack of cigarettes smoked. Tobacco smokers have decreased intake and absorption of vitamin C, as well as increased metabolic enzyme activity, both of which lead to a poorer vitamin C status. Other micronutrients are also depleted in smokers.

Recommended Dietary Allowances (RDAs) for Vitamin C in the United States and Canada

Age	Male (mg)	Female (mg)	Pregnancy (mg)	Lactation (mg)
0-6 months	40	40		
7-12 months	50	50		
1-3 years	15	15		
4-8 years	25	25		

9-13 years	45	45		
14-18 years	75	65	80	115
19+ years	90	75	85	120

Chapter 2

Food Sources of Vitamin C

Natural sources of Vitamin C

Vitamin C is mainly found in fruits and vegetables.

SOURCE (Portion size)	VITAMIN C (mg)
FRUIT	
Cantaloupe (1/4 Medium)	60
Fresh grapefruit (1/2 fruit)	40
Honeydew Melon (1/8 Medium)	40
Kiwi (1 Medium)	75
Mango (1 Cup, sliced)	45
Orange (1 Medium)	70
Papaya (1 Cup, cubes)	85
Strawberries (1 Cup, sliced)	95

Tangerines or tangelos (1 Medium)	25
Watermelon (1 Cup)	15
JUICE	
Grapefruit (1/2 Cup)	35
Orange (1/2 Cup)	50
Apple (1/2 Cup)	50
Cranberry juice cocktail (1/2 Cup)	45
Grape (1/2 Cup)	120
VEGETABLES	
Asparagus, cooked (1/2 Cup)	10
Broccoli, cooked (1/2 Cup)	60
Brussels sprouts, cooked (1/2 Cup)	50
Cabbage	
Red, raw, chopped (1/2 Cup)	20
Red, cooked (1/2 Cup)	25
Raw, chopped (1/2 Cup	10

Cooked (1/2 Cup)	15
Cauliflower, raw or cooked (1/2 Cup)	25
Kale, cooked (1 cup)	55
Mustard greens, cooked (1 cup)	35
Pepper, red or green	
Raw (1/2 Cup)	65
Cooked (1/2 Cup)	50
Plantains, sliced, cooked (1 Cup)	15
Potato, baked (1 Medium)	25
Snow peas	
Fresh, cooked (1/2 Cup)	40
Frozen, cooked (1/2 Cup)	20
Sweet potato	
Baked (1 Medium)	30

Vacuum Can (1 Cup)	50
Canned, syrup-pack (1 Cup)	20
Tomato	
Raw (1/2 Cup)	15
Canned (1/2 Cup)	35
Juice (6 fluid oz)	35

Fruits and vegetables rich in Vitamin C

Rich fruit sources include cantaloupe, grapefruit, honeydew, kiwi, mango, orange, papaya, strawberries, tangelo, tangerine and watermelon. Fruit juices containing vitamin C in abundance include grapefruit and orange juices. Several fruit juices are fortified with vitamin C, including apple, cranberry and grape juices.

Rich vegetable sources of vitamin C include asparagus, broccoli, brussels sprouts, cabbage, cauliflower, kale, mustard greens, pepper (red or green), plantains, potatoes, snow peas, sweet potatoes and tomatoes and tomato juices.

Variables that affect vitamin C content of fruits and vegetables are harvesting season, duration of transport to the marketplace, period of storage and cooking practices.

Cooking methods that preserve Vitamin C content

- Vitamin C is heat sensitive, therefore boiling or placing it under extreme heat might destroy it.

- Mixing a variety of raw and cooked fresh fruits and vegetables can help avoid vitamin C loss due to heat.

- Vitamin C is also water soluble, meaning it dissolves in water, therefore soaking your vegetables and fruits for an extended period of time is not recommended.

- When we prepare vegetables, vitamin C dissolves in the broth, thus the broth should not be thrown away.

- Do not discard the surplus water after boiling vegetables; it is high in nutrients and may be utilized to make gravies, knead bread, or used to make refreshment drinks.

- Root vegetables such as potatoes, ginger, turnip, and carrots should be cooked with their skins on, and the skins should be removed after boiling. This allows nutrients to migrate to the center of the veggies, resulting in higher nutrient retention.

- When exposed to air, vitamin C decomposes quickly. As a result, fruits and vegetables should not be stored for an extended period of time. Also, don't peel fruits and vegetables too far ahead of time, and chop them into bigger pieces to expose them to less air to prevent the loss of vitamin C.

- Vegetables can lose up to 25% of their ascorbic acid when frozen. Canned storage causes vitamin C losses of up to 20% during the sterilization process. Dehydration reduces the ascorbic acid content of food by 10-15%.

- When preparing food using water. It's best to let it come to a boil before adding the veggies. You reduce the cooking time by doing so.

- Using Copper pans to cook is also known to reduce vitamin C content

- The process of adding bicarbonate to vegetables depletes the vitamin C concentration.

- Use water-saving cooking methods. One of the finest methods is to use a microwave or pressure cooker, which cook without water and have a fast cooking time.

- Because of the limited interaction with water at relatively moderate temperatures, steaming and microwaving preserved greater quantities of vitamin C than boiling. Using less cooking water and cooking for shorter periods of time should result in more vitamin C retention.

- Steaming is the most effective technique of preserving the vitamin C content in vegetables.

Dietary tips for maximizing Vitamin C absorption

- The best way to absorb vitamin C is to eat it in a raw state. You can drink freshly squeezed citrus juices, but avoid packaged brands, which sometimes include dangerous additives and additional sugar. Fruits and vegetables, whether fresh or frozen, can be equally healthy.

- Iron and vitamin C work together, with iron and vitamin C absorption improved by consuming iron-rich foods like spinach, lentils, and red meat, with vitamin C-rich meals or supplements. One of the reasons Orange juice being consumed with Cereals is a common practice due to its iron content aiding in vitamin C absorption.

- Vitamin C's effectiveness depends on its consumption. It's best taken on an empty stomach, as it doesn't require fat for absorption. It's best taken in the morning or 30 minutes before meals. Large single doses can cause gastrointestinal discomfort, especially for those with sensitive stomachs, and may cause cramps, gas, or diarrhea.

- Although vitamin C is a water-soluble vitamin, it is more easily absorbed when combined with healthy fats. So include a source of healthy fats in your vitamin C-rich meals or snacks, such as avocado, almonds, or olive oil.

- Blend vitamin C-rich foods into smoothies or yogurt. Adding spinach to most smoothies will not significantly alter the flavor and will provide a boost of vitamins and minerals.

- Consider splitting your daily intake into numerous smaller doses to keep a consistent amount of vitamin C in your body. This can aid to improve nutrient absorption and utilization.

- Hydration is crucial for efficient nutrient absorption, particularly vitamin C absorption. Drink enough water throughout the day to aid absorption and distribution of this essential vitamin.

Increasing your diet of vitamin C-rich foods should be a priority, but if you're still not achieving your daily requirements, try a milder vitamin C supplement created from whole food sources. There are various vitamin C powders on the market manufactured from dehydrated and powdered foods that enhance absorption while also providing a host of other nutrients.

However if you find that powdered or pill versions of vitamin C cause minimal gastrointestinal upset, a liposomal form may be more suitable. Liposomes are phospholipids that wrap vitamin C and shield it from the stomach and destruction. It is absorbed in the gut and straight into the circulation after passing through the stomach.

According to research, only around 30% of vitamin C in tablet form is absorbed, but up to 98% of liposomal vitamin C is absorbed. Alternatively, by supplementing vitamin C with cofactors, you can significantly enhance its absorption rate. Buffered ascorbic acid may also be appropriate for persons who have digestive issues while taking standard vitamin C supplements; buffered vitamin C is combined with magnesium, potassium, and calcium to minimize GI symptoms and allow for greater dosages.

Chapter 3

The Health Benefits of Vitamin C

Boosting the Immune System

Leukocytes, such as neutrophils and monocytes, aggressively collect vitamin C against a concentration gradient, resulting in levels that are 50-to 100-fold greater than plasma concentrations. These cells acquire maximum vitamin C concentrations with dietary intakes of 100 mg/day, but other bodily tissues presumably require larger intakes for saturation. Neutrophils collect vitamin C through SVCT2 and normally have intracellular levels of at least 1 mM.

Following oxidative burst activation, neutrophils can raise their intracellular content of vitamin C by non-specific absorption of the oxidized form, dehydroascorbate (DHA), via glucose transporters (GLUT). DHA is subsequently quickly converted to ascorbate intracellularly, yielding levels of around 10 mM. It is thought that the buildup of such high vitamin C concentrations suggests crucial roles inside these cells. The accumulation of millimolar concentrations of vitamin C in neutrophils, particularly after activation of their oxidative burst, is considered to shield these cells from oxidative damage.

The role of vitamin C in phagocyte function. Vitamin C has been demonstrated to: (a) boost neutrophil movement in response to chemo attractants (chemotaxis), (b) promote microbe engulfment (phagocytosis), and (c) stimulate reactive oxygen species (ROS) formation and microbe death, (d) Vitamin C promotes caspase-dependent apoptosis by increasing macrophage uptake and clearance and inhibiting necrosis, particularly NETosis, so assisting in the resolution of the inflammatory reaction and minimizing damage to tissue.

Vitamin C's antioxidant qualities allow it to protect lung cells against oxidants and oxidant-mediated damage produced by a variety of contaminants, heavy metals, pesticides, and xenobiotics.

Promoting Skin Health and Collagen Production

The major role of the skin is to act as a barrier against environmental assaults, and its distinctive structure reflects this. The skin is made up of two layers: the epidermal outer layer, which is highly cellular and serves as a barrier, and the inner dermal layer, which offers strength and flexibility as well as nutritional support to the epidermis. Normal skin contains high concentrations of vitamin C, with levels comparable to other body tissues and well above plasma concentrations, indicating active accumulation from the circulation.

This vitamin C supports important and well-known functions, such as stimulating collagen synthesis and assisting in antioxidant protection against UV-induced photodamage.

A number of well-conducted intervention studies have found that eating fruits and vegetables is connected with better skin health. The active component in the fruits and vegetables responsible for the reported benefit has not been discovered, and the impact is likely to be multifactorial, despite the fact that vitamin C status is directly related to fruit and vegetable intake.

Vitamin C can help to reduce the signs of aging in human skin. A lot of research corroborates this, albeit measuring skin changes is difficult. Some research incorporates objective measurements of collagen deposition and wrinkle depth. The use of Vitamin C to the skin promotes wound healing and reduces the creation of raised scars. This has been proven in several clinical trials on people and animals.

Vitamin C works as a cofactor for the proline and lysine hydroxylases, which maintain the tertiary structure of the collagen molecule, and it also increases collagen gene expression. Collagen synthesis in the skin is primarily carried out by fibroblasts in the dermis, culminating in the creation of the basement membrane and dermal collagen matrix. The collagen hydroxylase enzymes' dependency on vitamin C has been confirmed in a number of in vitro investigations involving fibroblast cells, with both lower overall synthesis and decreased crosslinking when vitamin C is missing. Because the amount of collagen generated might vary very little, measuring the activity of the hydroxylases in vivo is much more challenging.

Rather, animal investigations with the vitamin-C-deficient GULO mice show that the stability of produced collagen fluctuates with vitamin C availability, ruling out the stabilizing function of the collagen crosslinks created by the hydroxylases. Vitamin C not only stabilizes the collagen molecule by hydroxylation, but it also increases fibroblast collagen mRNA synthesis.

As a consequence of study into the significance of vitamin C in skin health, the following information is now accessible. Skin fibroblasts are completely dependent on vitamin C for collagen production and dermal collagen/elastin balance control. This dependence may be demonstrated in vitro using grown cells. Additionally, vitamin C supplementation increased collagen production in vivo.

Skin Keratinocytes may collect significant levels of vitamin C, which, when combined with vitamin E, protects against UV irradiation. This information is derived from in vitro research with cultured cells, with additional data from animal and human investigations. Vitamin C regulates gene expression of antioxidant enzymes, the structure and accumulation of phospholipids, and the creation of the stratum corneum and epithelial differentiation in general, according to studies on keratinocytes in culture.

The delivery of vitamin C into the skin by topical application remains difficult. Although some human studies have demonstrated a favorable benefit in terms of UV irradiation protection, the most effective formulations comprise both vitamins C and E, as well as a delivery vehicle.

Antioxidant Properties and Protection from Free Radicals

Vitamin C is a powerful antioxidant that may neutralize and eliminate oxidants present in pollution and after exposure to UV radiation. This action appears to be especially important in the epidermis, which has the highest concentration of vitamin C in the skin. However, vitamin C is only one component of an antioxidant defense system that also includes enzymatic defenses (catalase, glutathione peroxidase, and superoxide dismutase) and non-enzymatic defenses (vitamin E, glutathione, uric acid, and other putative antioxidants such as carotenoids). The majority of intervention studies employed a combination of these substances to test the potential of antioxidants to prevent oxidative damage to skin.

Yet because vitamin C is an electron donor and a reducing agent, the majority of its physiological and biochemical activities are ascribed to this, which is why it is regarded as such a potent antioxidant. And vitamin C has a distinguishing characteristic that most other compounds do not. Molecules require a full outer shell of electrons to be stable; when these electrons are lost, they become unstable and extremely reactive (i.e., they form free radicals). The exception to this rule is vitamin C. When vitamin C loses an electron, it stays very stable, making it one of the body's finest free radical scavengers and hence a potent antioxidant.

As previously stated, vitamin C may be oxidized by a variety of species that may be implicated in human diseases. There are various types of organisms that acquire electrons and are reduced by vitamin C:

1. Compounds containing unpaired electrons (radicals), such as oxygen radicals (superoxide, hydroxyl radicals, peroxyl radicals), sulfur radicals, and nitrogen-oxygen radicals. These molecules, with the exception of sulfur radicals, are sometimes referred to as reactive oxygen species and reactive nitrogen species.

2. Reactive but non-radical chemicals, such as hypochlorous acid, nitrosamines and other nitrosating substances, nitrous acid-related compounds, and ozone.

3. Compounds created by combining the preceding two groups and then reacting with vitamin C. The creation of the alpha tocopheroxyl radical, which occurs when exogenous radical oxidants interact with alpha tocopherol in low-density lipoprotein (LDL), is one example. Ascorbate can convert the radical back to alpha tocopherol.

4. Iron and copper-mediated transition metal processes. For example, reduction of iron by ascorbate might result in the creation of additional radicals via Fenton chemistry. Reduced iron, on the other hand, might be an endpoint reaction: for example, reduced iron may be the favored state for intestinal absorption.

Antioxidant action in Lipids

Lipids, particularly membrane lipids and lipids found in circulating lipoproteins such as low-density lipoprotein (LDL), can interact with reactive oxygen species, resulting in lipid peroxidation. Once formed, lipid peroxides can react with oxygen to produce extremely reactive peroxyl radicals. The synthesis of lipid hydroperoxides can continue indefinitely, a process known as radical propagation. Ascorbate can decrease early or ongoing lipid peroxidation by reducing the starting reactive oxygen species. Proteins, like lipids, can undergo radical propagation, resulting in the production of new reactive species. Ascorbate can reduce protein or amino acid oxidation and radical propagation by lowering radical initiators.

Antioxidant action in DNA

Reactive nitrogen species, some of which can be produced from nitrosamines, can also damage DNA. Nitric oxide radicals and similar chemicals, for example, can induce DNA strand breakage and point mutations. Ascorbate should be able to reduce DNA damage by directly reducing radical species, lowering the generation of reactive species such lipid hydroperoxides, or avoiding radical assault on proteins that repair DNA. Ascorbate, as an antioxidant, can inhibit nitrosamine production, hence preventing the creation of some reactive nitrogen species. Ascorbate's ability to suppress mutagenesis activity becomes less effective once nitrosamines produce reactive nitrogen species. Ascorbate therefore decreases a wide range of oxidant species; reactions generating these species may occur in a number of cell compartments, altering lipids, proteins, and DNA, and some of these reaction products may be quantified with and without ascorbate.

Antioxidant action in Endothelial Function

Vitamin C may boost endothelial nitric oxide (NO) generation by shielding it from oxidation. Vitamin C and the other antioxidant vitamin, vitamin E, appear to improve vascular endothelial function in both healthy and cardiovascular disease patients. According to some data, increasing vascular oxidative stress plays a role in the pathogenesis of endothelial dysfunction and hypertension. Low plasma vitamin C levels have been linked to hypertension and reduced endothelial function.

Vitamin C, which is abundant in fruits and vegetables, may protect NO from oxidation and improve endothelial function. This might explain some of the cardiovascular-protective benefits of fruits and vegetables.

Antioxidant action in Gastric Function

Vitamin C may help quench reactive oxygen metabolites in the stomach or duodenum, preventing the development of carcinogenic N-nitroso compounds. Gastric cancer has been related to nitrosamines. Vitamin C treatment can reduce the formation of nitrosamines in the gastrointestinal system. A high dietary vitamin C consumption is associated with a lower incidence of stomach cancer.

Antioxidant action in the Skin

When combined with vitamin E, vitamin C is very efficient at reducing oxidative damage to the skin. This is consistent with its recognized role as an oxidized vitamin E regenerator, successfully recycling this crucial lipid-soluble radical scavenger and reducing oxidative damage to cell membrane components.

Many diseases that are considered to be caused or aggravated by oxidant stress are associated with low plasma and tissue vitamin C concentrations. Smoking and diabetes mellitus are the two most frequent prooxidant conditions associated with low plasma vitamin C concentrations.

Wound Healing and Tissue Repair

Wound healing is a complicated process that consists of three major sequential and overlapping stages: inflammation, new tissue creation, and remodeling.

The most striking and consistent impact of vitamin C on skin health is its positive influence on wound healing. This is due to its cofactor role in collagen formation, with poor wound healing being an early sign of hypovitaminosis C. Because of local inflammation and the needs of increased collagen formation, vitamin C turnover at wound sites implies that supplementation is important, and both topical administration and increased food intake have been found to be effective.

Both vitamin C and vitamin E supplementation enhanced the pace of wound healing in children with significant burns, and plasma vitamin C levels in smokers, abstaining smokers, and non-smokers were positively linked with the rate of wound healing.

However, it appears that the amount of the benefits of supplemented vitamin C consumption is, once again, contingent on the individual's baseline state, with any benefit being less evident if dietary intake is already adequate. However, the intricacy of the research and poor study population selection have frequently made it impossible to reach firm conclusions on the efficacy of nutritional therapies, as highlighted in a meta-analysis evaluating the effects of several treatments on ulcer healing.

A recent study found that topical administration of vitamin C in a silicone gel reduced persistent scar development in an Asian population.

Scurvy symptoms include wound dehiscence, poor wound healing, and tooth loosening, all of which lead to connective tissue abnormalities. Collagen offers structural strength to connective tissue. Vitamin C catalyzes the enzymatic posttranslational modification of procollagen, allowing collagen generating cells to create and release enough amounts of structurally normal collagen, hence enhancing connective tissue strength.

Enhancing Iron Absorption

It has long been known that Ascorbic Acid improves iron absorption, but with the advent of new methodologies to research iron absorption in recent years, it has become clear that Ascorbic Acid is the most effective promoter of dietary iron absorption.

Ascorbic acid's mechanism of action is typically linked to either its capacity to generate soluble iron complexes or its ability to decrease ferric to ferrous ions. Both methods lower the likelihood that iron ions will be tightly coupled to other ligands in the intestinal material, such as hydroxyl ions, preventing iron absorption. Thus, ascorbic acid will counteract the effect of ligands that bind iron ions and impede iron absorption.

Phytates and polyphenols are the most powerful dietary iron inhibitors known.

According to the research given above, Ascorbic Acid improves iron absorption from all types of meals, including those with no known inhibitor of nonheme iron absorption. They also demonstrate that the relative effect of Ascorbic Acid is greater when a meal contains potent inhibitors of iron absorption, such as phytates, but that more Ascorbic Acid is required in such a meal to counteract the inhibition of iron absorption, and that more Ascorbic Acid is required as the phytate content increases. More Ascorbic Acid is consequently required in a diet heavy in grains, legumes, and vegetables to balance their greater phytate and tannin content.

There is no doubt that Ascorbic Acid is extremely important for iron absorption. Even if iron may be absorbed from the food without Ascorbic Acid, the impact is so strong and consistent that it must be regarded as a physiological element that is required for dietary iron absorption.

Nonheme iron accounts for more than 90% of dietary iron. Its absorbability is determined by the balance of variables that promote and impede absorption. Ascorbic acid is the most powerful booster, and this is true for both natural and manufactured Ascorbic Acid.

The boosting impact is substantially dose dependent (log dose/effect) and varies across meals, most likely due to the varied inhibitor content of the meals.

Ascorbic Acid also enhances iron absorption from simple meals with no known inhibitors, most likely through impairing the formation of inaccessible iron complexes with ligands typically present in the gastrointestinal lumen. However only if ascorbic acid is present in the meal will it be effective.

Chapter 4

Vitamin C and Disease Prevention

Cardiovascular Health and Reducing the Risk of Heart Disease

Vitamin C has been shown to prevent apoptosis by inhibiting the activity of inflammatory cytokines and oxidized Low Density Lipoprotein (LDL) in both cultured endothelial cells and patients with congestive heart failure, where treatment with vitamin C reduced the release of microparticles derived from endothelial cells.

Indeed, vitamin C increases Nitric Oxide (NO) synthase activity by keeping tetrahydrobiopterin, an important cofactor for the enzyme, in its reduced and active state, which is ordinarily hindered by reactive oxygen species (ROS) that oxidize and so deplete the cofactor. Vitamin C may indirectly protect the vascular endothelium by boosting NO production through its activities, which include smooth muscle cell relaxation, downstream vasodilation, and inhibition of the effects of pro-inflammatory cytokines and adhesion molecules that are significant in atherosclerosis. However many studies has shown Vitamin C does not have a direct significant effect on Cardiovascular diseases but enough intake of Vitamin C may mitigate the risks and effects

Eye Health and Prevention of Age-Related Macular Degeneration

The eye includes a high quantity of ascorbate, which protects it against free radical damage caused by photolysis, which can lead to cataracts and macular degeneration. The role of vitamin C in the prevention of ocular diseases has been studied, and it has been shown that ascorbate influences the development of cataracts and that combining ascorbate with other antioxidant vitamins and minerals slows the progression of advanced age-related macular degeneration and loss of visual acuity in people who have symptoms of this disease.

Two case-control studies found that taking more than 300 mg of vitamin C per day lowered the incidence of cataract by 70-75%. Furthermore, plasma ascorbate concentrations greater than 90 mol/L were linked to a 71% decreased incidence of cataract. Vitamin C consumption also influences ascorbate concentrations in the lens. Consumption of 150 to 250 mg per day may saturate ocular tissues.

The usefulness of vitamin C as a therapy for diabetic retinopathy has also been investigated, although further research is needed to confirm that it has a substantial impact on its progression.

Role in cancer prevention

Many cancer patients undergoing severe chemotherapy are deficient in vitamin C. Because vitamin C boosts the development and activation of immune cells, it is possible that supplementation might help such patients' immunity. In acute myeloid leukemia patients, the strongest evidence of a beneficial impact is shown in combination with decitabine.

Furthermore, we demonstrated in preclinical investigations that vitamin C plays a significant role in the immune system by stimulating the development and/or activation of immune cells such as T-lymphocytes and natural killer cells, which fight infections and cancer cells.

It was discovered that many patients receiving intense chemotherapy and stem cell transplants for hematological malignancies have low vitamin C plasma concentrations in earlier vitamin C studies.

This might be due to these individuals' inadequate food intake or an increased requirement for vitamin C in tumor cells or in immune cells. Other studies found that low vitamin C plasma levels in individuals with various forms of advanced cancer were related with poorer survival.

Patients undergoing extensive chemotherapy and/or stem cell transplants are vulnerable to infection problems. Boosting their immune system with vitamin C to expedite immunological recovery and hence avoid viral problems is appealing because vitamin C is inexpensive and widely accessible.

Even at large doses of intravenous vitamin C supplementation, treatment is expected to be safe, with essentially no significant adverse effects and few moderate side effects. There is also no evidence that vitamin C supplementation hastens cancer progression.

Daily supplementation with 14 vitamins and 12 minerals has been shown to reduce esophageal and gastric cancer mortality and rates of total cancer.

Because of its pro-oxidant activity, vitamin C may also act as a cancer cell killer. The effective concentration of vitamin C necessary to mediate cancer death is simpler to attain by intravenous injection than via oral administration. Among the potential reasons include stimulatory effects on apoptotic pathways, faster pro-oxidant damage that tumor cells cannot repair, and enhanced oxidation of ascorbate to the unstable metabolite dehydroascorbic acid (DHA), which can be lethal to tumor cells.

Extracellular H_2O_2 production, with the ascorbate radical as an intermediary, is required for cancer cell death. H_2O_2 produced by pharmaceutical ascorbate doses diffuses into cells and kills tumor cells in minutes. H_2O_2 inside cells may induce DNA and mitochondrial breaks, and mitochondria in some cancer cells may be more sensitive to H2O2. Among other anti-cancer strategies, ascorbic acid has previously been postulated to play a function in boosting collagen production and blocking hyaluronidase. These methods are thought to limit cancer spread by thickening the extracellular matrix, resulting in tumor walling.

A randomized, placebo-controlled clinical trial in which a large dose of vitamin C was administered orally to advanced cancer patients yielded inconclusive findings, throwing doubt on vitamin C's usefulness in cancer treatment. Because of the disagreement surrounding the vitamin C-cancer association and the lack of a confirmed molecular basis for its therapeutic activity, further study is needed to assess the practicality of employing vitamin C in clinical cancer therapy or prevention.

Reducing the Risk of Respiratory Infections

Vitamin C is largely found in the respiratory tract's epithelial lining, where it acts as an immunostimulant, alleviating symptoms of upper respiratory tract infections. By increasing numerous immune cell activities, vitamin C appears to be capable of both preventing and treating respiratory and systemic infections. Prophylactic infection prevention necessitates appropriate, if not saturating, plasma levels of vitamin C (i.e., 100-200 mg/day), which maximize cell and tissue levels. To compensate for the increased metabolic requirement, treatment of established illnesses necessitates much greater (gram) dosages of the vitamin.

Viral and bacterial infections have the potential to lower vitamin C levels because they create reactive oxygen and nitrogen species via leukocyte activation, which leads to the oxidation of extracellular vitamin C. Changes in vitamin C metabolism caused by respiratory infections imply that vitamin C may be useful to persons suffering from pneumonia.

According to recent data, individuals with Chronic Respiratory Disease had a much lower average daily vitamin C consumption than healthy volunteers. So when compared to healthy controls, Chronic Obstructive Pulmonary Disease (COPD) patients had lower vitamin C levels in their blood and diet.

In a study on the effects of vitamin C on respiratory infections, reported flu and cold symptoms in the test group decreased by 85% compared to the control group following megadose Vitamin C administration. It was shown that supplementing asthmatic patients with a blend of vitamin C-containing antioxidants for two months reduced levels of high sensitivity C reactive protein (CRP) and malondialdehyde (MDA) in their blood.

Even though Vitamin C might not be able to cure respiratory infections, its administration has shown to reduce the effects of respiratory infections and compensate for the nutrients deficiency in treatment of these infections.

Chapter 5

Vitamin C and Mental Well-being

Role in Reducing Stress and Anxiety

This vitamin is required for glucocorticoid production because ascorbic acid is a cofactor for enzymes found in the adrenal cortex that participate in the glucocorticoid biosynthesis pathway. Ascorbate, for example, is a cofactor for 11-hydroxylase, boosting to a modest degree the conversion of 11-deoxycortisol to cortisol and maintaining cortisol tone under physiological settings. High amounts of ascorbic acid in the adrenal gland, as well as its release in reaction to ACTH, show that ascorbic acid plays an essential role in the stress response.

In line with this, studies on the depletion of ascorbate stores in the adrenal gland following systemic ACTH administration to hypophysectomized rats have shown that ascorbate release occurs before corticosteroid release, implying that under stress, the adrenal gland must first release the amount of ascorbate it has before steroid synthesis (or release) can begin.

Interestingly, several clinical trials found that ascorbic acid might reduce stress hormone levels and subjective sensations of stress. For example, ascorbic acid (3 g/day for 5 days) attenuated the rise in cortisol levels induced by exogenous ACTH, indicating that ascorbic acid can be utilized to restrict the effects of stress hormones.

The depressed symptoms generated by ACTH treatment in a 5-year-old child with hepatitis B were restored by intravenous ascorbic acid therapy (50 mg/kg/day for 2 weeks). A randomized clinical experiment employing sustained-release of a high dosage of ascorbic acid (3 × 1000 mg/day for 14 days) lowered the subjective reaction to psychological stress in the trier social stress test.

Brain Health and Cognitive Function

Vitamin C appears to be allowed to penetrate numerous brain cell lines, increasing neurotransmission and influencing activities such as learning, memory, and motility.

It is generally understood that the primary function of intracellular ascorbic acid in the brain is cell antioxidant defense. However, vitamin C has several non-antioxidant roles in the central nervous system (CNS). It is an enzymatic cofactor in the manufacture of molecules such as collagen, carnitine, tyrosine, and peptide hormones. Ascorbic acid has also been shown to induce the synthesis of myelin in Schwann cells.

The brain is an organ that is particularly vulnerable to oxidative stress and free radical activity, which is associated with high quantities of unsaturated fatty acids and a rapid rate of cell metabolism. Ascorbic acid, as an antioxidant, works directly by scavenging reactive oxygen and nitrogen species created during normal cell metabolism. In vivo investigations revealed that ascorbate had the potential to inactivate superoxide radicals, a significant consequence of mitochondrial neuron rapid metabolism. In light of these data, vitamin C is thought to be a significant neuroprotective agent.

Depression Prevention and Mood Enhancement

Depression is a sign of various vitamin deficiencies, one of which is vitamin C, which is renowned for its antidepressant properties. Vitamin C is a well-known modulator of neurotransmitter production. It acts as a cofactor for dopamine hydroxylase in the conversion of dopamine to norepinephrine (NE), which is vital in mood control. A chronic deficiency of vitamin C causes a drop in NE levels. Vitamin C is also a cofactor for the tryptophan-5-hydroxylase enzyme, which is essential for the conversion of tryptophan to 5-hydroxytryptophan in the creation of serotonin, and its absence contributes to depression.

Sleep Quality and Vitamin C's Impact

According to studies, consumers use nutritional supplements for a variety of reasons, including illness prevention, improved immune function, energy, memory, and focus, and improved sleep health. Sleep is an essential component of newborn, child, and adolescent health and development. Sleep, together with nutrition and exercise, is a crucial predictor of human physical and mental well-being.

To have a restorative effect on the body, sleep must be of adequate quality and duration, which means that the following factors must be considered: the total amount of sleep obtained per 24 h, the ease of falling asleep and returning to sleep, the placement of sleep within the 24 h day, the ability to maintain attentive wakefulness, and, finally, the subjective assessment of "good" or "bad" sleep.

The relationship of many different nutrients with sleep symptoms such as difficulty falling asleep, sleep maintenance difficulties, poor sleep quality, non-restorative sleep and increased daytime sleepiness, and sleep duration has mostly been studied in small trials or cross-sectional studies in healthy adults. Fruits and vegetables are the primary dietary sources of vitamin C, and their consumption is related with higher levels of plasma antioxidants. People who slept for a lengthy period of time (more than 8 hours per day) had greater plasma vitamin C levels than reference sleepers. This might be explained by the use of different diets or the disparity between the biomarkers used to measure long-term dietary consumption and the diet intake measured by a four-day food diary.

It should be noted that melancholy, anxiety disorders, and psychosocial stress, which are psychological causes of sleeplessness, are linked to oxidative damage. Although the neurobiological mechanism underlying ascorbic acid's neuroprotective properties is not fully understood, both preclinical and clinical evidence has demonstrated its beneficial effects on stress-related diseases such as depression and anxiety. It is highly possible that vitamin C intake, which has an antidepressant effect and boosts mood, alleviates insomnia symptoms.

The existing research suggests that vitamin C is vital for sleep not only in healthy persons but also in cancer patients. Increased use of this antioxidant may assist to extend sleep duration, minimize sleep disruptions, alleviate movement problems, and prevent the hazardous effects of sleep apnea. Current studies findings also suggest that taking Vitamin C protects against chronic sleep deprivation-induced short- and long-term memory deficits.

Chapter 6

Vitamin C Deficiency and Supplements

Vitamin C Deficiency and its Symptoms

Scurvy is caused by a lack of vitamin C. Scurvy symptoms include muscle weakness, swollen and bleeding gums, tooth loss, petechial hemorrhaging, spontaneous ecchymoses, anemia, impaired wound healing, hyperkeratosis, weakness, myalgia, arthralgia, and weight loss (there can also be a paradoxical weight increase due to swelling), and weight loss (there can also be a paradoxical weight increase due to swelling). Dyspnea might also be noted. Scurvy can be lethal, and rapid death has happened as a result of a cerebral/myocardial hemorrhage or pneumonia.

Classical and more modern investigations of scurvy in natural environments have typically found that behavioral indications such as listlessness, lassitude, weakness, and reluctance to effort contribute to the clinical picture of scurvy.

Collagen production is hampered and connective tissues are weakened as vitamin C deficiency continues, resulting in petechiae, ecchymoses, purpura, joint discomfort, poor wound healing, hyperkeratosis, and corkscrew hairs. Scurvy symptoms include depression, swollen and bleeding gums, and tooth loosening or loss owing to tissue and capillary fragility. Iron deficiency anemia can also arise as a result of increased bleeding and decreased nonheme iron absorption as a result of inadequate vitamin C consumption. Bone disease can occur in youngsters. Scurvy is lethal if it is not treated.

Populations at Risk of Deficiency

Dietary intake of vitamin C is a critical driver of body state, with the quantity taken and frequency of consumption associated with plasma status and the prevalence of insufficiency.

Geographic factors and agricultural techniques influence the production and consumption of staple foods in low and middle-income countries (LMICs), which can have a significant impact on vitamin C intake. Countries where rice and millet are staple foods, for example (as in Asia and portions of Africa), have lower vitamin C consumption.

Vitamin C consumption may be greater in several African and Latin American countries where yams and sweet potatoes are staple foods. However, the vitamin C concentration in food might vary depending on when it is harvested, how it is transported and stored, and how it is prepared. For example, differing processing procedures dramatically diminish the vitamin C content of some staple foods, such as cassava, which might lead to discrepancies in estimated vitamin C consumption. Cooking can degrade vitamin C since it is heat-labile; the poorer vitamin C status of Indians and Malays in Singapore is assumed to be attributable in part to its breakdown by longer cooking.

Given that most individuals acquire their vitamin C from fresh fruits and vegetables, it's not unexpected that there have been reports of seasonal changes in vitamin C status. However, research in England and China have found that vitamin C status is highest in winter and lowest in fall. This is most likely due to the types or amounts of vitamin C-rich foods ingested throughout the winter. In northern India, similar tendencies were seen; however, in southern India, the winter months were linked with a greater frequency of insufficiency.

Environmental cigarette smoke exposure is linked to vitamin C deficiency in both nonsmokers and children. Despite equal dietary intakes of vitamin C, it was discovered that the vitamin C status of passive smokers was considerably lower than that of non-exposed nonsmokers. Hypovitaminosis C was seen in 12% of passive smokers but not in nonsmokers who had never smoked. Females tend to have higher vitamin C status and a lower frequency of insufficiency in high-income environments than males.

A number of studies have found that, within the same research group, older age is related with an increased prevalence of vitamin C insufficiency, particularly in males, and that older men had lower vitamin C consumption than older women. Bodyweight, as well as BMI, waist circumference, and waist-to-hip ratio, are widely established to have a substantial relationship with vitamin C status. Pearson, a researcher, discovered that those who had hypovitaminosis C had considerably greater weight, BMI, and waist circumference. Decreased vitamin C status in persons with the greatest body mass index may be attributable in part to a decreased dietary intake of the vitamin. In support of this, those with the greatest fat intake had poorer vitamin C status.

Noncommunicable diseases such as cardiovascular diseases (e.g., strokes, coronary artery disease, and hypertension), congestive heart failure, malignancy, chronic inflammatory states (e.g., rheumatoid arthritis), metabolic disorders (e.g., diabetes), and cataracts are all linked to vitamin C deficiency. It should also be mentioned that persons with low vitamin C status are more likely to develop vitamin C deficiency, and once depleted, greater than recommended vitamin C doses are necessary to adequately replenish them.

Choosing the Right Vitamin C Supplement

When looking for a vitamin C supplement, evaluate the quality, dosage, and price. You should also consider the type of supplement you desire, such as chewable pills or a powder.

Quality

Investigate a brand's ingredient source and seek for suppliers who adhere to the current Good Manufacturing Practices specified by the Food and Drug Administration (FDA). To confirm that a product includes what it claims to contain, search for one that has been evaluated by a third-party agency, such as USP, Consumer Lab, or NSF International.

Finally, it's worth checking the ingredient list and selecting a product that doesn't include any artificial additives or preservatives. Similarly, if you're attempting to cut back on added sugar, you should avoid sweetened supplements.

Ingredients

Choose items that are properly labeled and include safe and high-quality components. They should also affirm that they are pesticide, heavy metal, and mold free.

Dosage

Dosage is a crucial factor because vitamin C supplements come in a variety of dosages. It is suggested that most healthy men and women ingest 90 mg and 75 mg of vitamin C per day, respectively.

Some people, however, may benefit from a greater dose of vitamin C. If this is the case, finding a concentrated supplement may be more cost effective and handy. You won't have to take many servings of a lower dosage choice this way.

High doses of 1,000 mg or more are often unneeded and may contribute to undesired side effects. Only take excessive amounts if your doctor advises you to.

Price

Some professional-grade products might be pricey, but remember that a greater price does not always imply a superior quality. There are always several high-quality alternatives available at a variety of pricing points.

Form

Vitamin C supplements come in a variety of formats, including liquids, pills that can be chewed, tablets that can be swallowed and in powdered form.

If you want to take a tablet, look into encapsulated vitamin C pills. If you dislike ingesting pills or wish to incorporate the supplement with liquids, you should get a liquid or powdered formulation.

Testing by a third party

Selects items that must have been tested for pollutants by a third party.

Safety guidelines and potential side effects

People who use more than 1,000 mg of vitamin C per day may have stomach discomfort, diarrhea, and gas. According to the National Library of Medicine, vitamin C via intravenous administration might cause headaches, dizziness, and flushing. Migraine can occur with a daily intake of 6 g. It also states that consuming a lot of vitamin C might raise your chances of getting kidney stones. It also adds that if a person has a blood problem, such as sickle cell disease, thalassemia, or hemochromatosis, doctors may not prescribe vitamin C supplementation.

Some drugs, such as chemotherapy and radiation, may interact with vitamin C. According to the National Institutes of Health (NIH), vitamin C has interacted with drugs used to reduce blood cholesterol levels. So before taking a vitamin C supplement, people should consult with their doctor to verify that it will not interfere with any existing prescriptions or health issues.

Chapter 7

Debunking Myths about Vitamin C

Separating fact from fiction

Most animals can produce vitamin C, however others have lost this capacity. Animals without vitamin C synthesis capacity have no evolutionary link to one another, meaning that several distinct mutations all result in the same trait. There is no discernible environmental effect. To this current time, no evolutionary explanation for the seemingly random loss of vitamin C synthesis capacity has been found. It is likely that some species have lost their capacity to manufacture vitamin C but have not been identified. Identification of all non-synthesizers might potentially improve pattern recognition, although thus far no such evidence exists.

Most tissues in humans and many animals contain high levels of vitamin C. However, for the known enzymatic effects of vitamin C, significantly lower amounts, potentially 1-2 orders of magnitude lower, are required.

Why are tissues so eager to absorb vitamin C ? One possible explanation is that sustaining concentrations well beyond the needed function may be an evolutionary protective or 'safety' role. If consumption was suddenly discontinued, enzymatic effects and deficiency would take time to emerge. Alternatively, intracellular accumulation at far greater concentrations than those required for enzymatic activity may imply that vitamin C has additional, as-yet undiscovered, roles. And only intravenous or parenteral dosing of ascorbate results in high concentrations (>5 mM vs. lM) of vitamin C in extracellular fluid.

At pharmacological quantities, ascorbate is known to create hydrogen peroxide.

In humans, the adrenal gland quickly releases/secretes ascorbate in response to the tropic hormone Adrenocorticotropic hormone (ACTH).

Ascorbate is also produced by the testes and the ovary in mammals. In the stomach, ascorbate is also secreted.

Scurvy is unavoidably caused by a lack of vitamin C. Nonetheless, scurvy cannot be treated without vitamin C.

The manner of administration appears to be a key element in the efficacy of vitamin C therapy. Intravenous delivery was employed in trials with good results, whereas oral administration was used in research with negative results. This shows that the vitamin C levels attained with oral supplementation may be insufficient to provide an impact, or that vitamin C is not absorbed from the gastrointestinal system.

Common misconceptions about Vitamin C

Vitamin C, by definition, is an electron donor, also known as an antioxidant. However, the commonly held belief that vitamin C has a vital antioxidant function in humans is unsubstantiated. To present, vitamin C supplementation has demonstrated little effect in illness states thought to be induced or exacerbated by oxidant stress.

Vitamin C is useful in the prevention and treatment of the common cold. Prophylactic vitamin C supplementation had no effect on the incidence of common cold in the general population, but had a small effect on the duration (by 8% in adults, 13% in children) and intensity of cold symptoms.

Because vitamin C stimulates iron absorption, some people claimed that taking vitamin C supplements was harmful to those who had iron excess or hemochromatosis. High plasma ascorbate levels, on the other hand, protect against oxidative damage caused by excess iron in animals and humans with iron overload. Indeed, the prescription for these people is to decrease their iron consumption rather than avoid ascorbate.

The consumption of large doses of vitamin C supplements has also been occasionally associated with skin rash, heartburn, nausea, and diarrhea. These are usually the result of the formulation of the vitamin C tablets but may also be caused by excessive consumption of vitamin C in a short period of time. Large doses of vitamin C have been anecdotally associated with vitamin B12 deficiency and systemic conditioning (also known as "rebound scurvy"), conditions that have never been documented clinically. Patients with glucose-6-phosphate dehydrogenase (G6PD) deficiency have also been cautioned against taking vitamin C supplements, due to reports of hemolytic anemia that have also not been substantiated.

The production of kidney stones is another widely stated concern of ascorbate supplementation, as oxalate is a byproduct of dehydroascorbic acid degradation. The data relating ascorbate supplement consumption and the occurrence of kidney stones in otherwise healthy people is conflicting. Excessive vitamin C oxidation would be required to produce large quantities of oxalate from ascorbate, however the mechanism underlying this oxidation has not been investigated. Studies that imply an elevated risk found it in those who took more than 1000 mg of vitamin C per day, significantly more than the amount that may be gained through diet. Without more research, patients with renal illness or a history of kidney stones should avoid taking significant quantities of vitamin C supplements. Unfortunately, this has led practitioners to advise dialysis patients to significantly limit their vitamin C usage, resulting in deficits.

Chapter 8

Incorporating Vitamin C into Your Lifestyle

Practical Tips for Increasing Vitamin C Intake

Fortunately, many of the finest vitamin C dietary sources, such as fruits and vegetables, are typically ingested uncooked. A daily intake of five different fruits and vegetables can give more than 200 mg of vitamin C. Vitamin C supplements often include ascorbic acid, which has the same bioavailability as naturally occurring ascorbic acid in foods like orange juice and broccoli.

Sodium ascorbate, calcium ascorbate, other mineral ascorbates, ascorbic acid with bioflavonoids, and combination products such as Ester-C, which combines calcium ascorbate, dehydroascorbate, calcium threonate, xylonate, and lyxonate, are examples of vitamin C supplements.

Vitamin C is heat sensitive, therefore boiling, steaming, or placing it under extreme heat might destroy it. The best methods for preserving vitamin A are stir-frying or blanching.

Eating a variety of raw and cooked fresh fruits and vegetables can help avoid vitamin C loss due to heat.

Choose seasonal fruits and vegetables. Seasonal food contains the most vitamin C. If you can't get food in season, go for frozen fruits and vegetables, which are often produced and frozen at optimum freshness.

Drink your vitamin C. If you prefer to drink your vitamin C rather than eat it, juices (orange, mixed fruit, tomato) or smoothies might help.

Between meals, snack on fruits and vegetables. If you want to get additional vitamin C, nibble on these extra-rich sources. A tasty vitamin C-rich snack is cherry tomatoes or bell peppers.

Recipes and Meal Ideas Rich in Vitamin C

Fruits salad containing ingredients of vitamin c rich fruits such as orange, lemon, guava, mango, pineapple, papaya, strawberry, kiwi and grape fruit.

Vegetables salad containing ingredients of vitamin c rich vegetables such as cabbage, bell peppers, chili peppers, broccoli, cantaloupe, cauliflower, tomatoes persimmon, potato, kale, spinach and brussel sprouts.

Smoothies containing pineapple, mango, strawberry, guava, tomatoes, lemon and guava.

Juices rich in orange, lemon, mango, guava, strawberry and pineapple

Conclusion

In concluding our exploration of "Everything You Need to Know about Vitamin C," it becomes evident that this humble vitamin plays a profound role in sustaining our overall well-being. From its historical discovery to its essential functions within the body, Vitamin C has earned its status as a vital nutrient with far-reaching implications for health.

Throughout this journey, we delved into the multifaceted benefits of Vitamin C, ranging from its potent antioxidant properties combating oxidative stress to its crucial role in collagen synthesis for skin health. We navigated the landscape of recommended daily allowances, emphasizing the significance of maintaining a balanced diet rich in natural sources of this essential vitamin.

As we uncovered the potential consequences of Vitamin C deficiency and insufficiency, it became apparent that awareness and proactive measures are fundamental in preventing associated health issues, such as scurvy. We explored the realm of supplements, scrutinizing their benefits and offering guidelines for optimal usage while acknowledging the importance of diverse dietary sources.

In our exploration of cooking and storage tips, we learned that preserving Vitamin C's potency is not only possible but crucial for reaping its benefits. By dispelling myths and presenting evidence-based facts, we sought to empower readers with accurate information, fostering a deeper understanding of this critical nutrient.

Special considerations were not overlooked, as we examined the impact of Vitamin C on different demographics.

In essence, this comprehensive guide aims to serve as a beacon of knowledge, illuminating the path towards a healthier, Vitamin C-enriched life. As we bid farewell, let us carry forward the wisdom gleaned from these pages, making informed choices that nurture our bodies and minds. May the journey toward optimal health be as vibrant and robust as the benefits provided by Vitamin C itself.